**PREGNANCY AND INFANTS:
MEDICAL, PSYCHOLOGICAL AND SOCIAL ISSUES**

ACUTE APPENDICITIS IN PREGNANCY

PREGNANCY AND INFANTS: MEDICAL, PSYCHOLOGICAL AND SOCIAL ISSUES

Additional books in this series can be found on Nova's website under the Series tab.

PREGNANCY AND INFANTS:
MEDICAL, PSYCHOLOGICAL AND SOCIAL ISSUES

ACUTE APPENDICITIS IN PREGNANCY

GORAN AUGUSTIN
AND
MATE MAJEROVIĆ

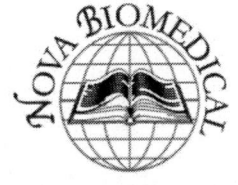

Nova Biomedical Books
New York

Copyright © 2011 by Nova Science Publishers, Inc.

All rights reserved. No part of this book may be reproduced, stored in a retrieval system or transmitted in any form or by any means: electronic, electrostatic, magnetic, tape, mechanical photocopying, recording or otherwise without the written permission of the Publisher.

For permission to use material from this book please contact us:
Telephone 631-231-7269; Fax 631-231-8175
Web Site: http://www.novapublishers.com

NOTICE TO THE READER

The Publisher has taken reasonable care in the preparation of this book, but makes no expressed or implied warranty of any kind and assumes no responsibility for any errors or omissions. No liability is assumed for incidental or consequential damages in connection with or arising out of information contained in this book. The Publisher shall not be liable for any special, consequential, or exemplary damages resulting, in whole or in part, from the readers' use of, or reliance upon, this material. Any parts of this book based on government reports are so indicated and copyright is claimed for those parts to the extent applicable to compilations of such works.

Independent verification should be sought for any data, advice or recommendations contained in this book. In addition, no responsibility is assumed by the publisher for any injury and/or damage to persons or property arising from any methods, products, instructions, ideas or otherwise contained in this publication.

This publication is designed to provide accurate and authoritative information with regard to the subject matter covered herein. It is sold with the clear understanding that the Publisher is not engaged in rendering legal or any other professional services. If legal or any other expert assistance is required, the services of a competent person should be sought. FROM A DECLARATION OF PARTICIPANTS JOINTLY ADOPTED BY A COMMITTEE OF THE AMERICAN BAR ASSOCIATION AND A COMMITTEE OF PUBLISHERS.
Additional color graphics may be available in the e-book version of this book.

Library of Congress Cataloging-in-Publication Data

Augustin, Goran.
Acute appendicitis in pregnancy / Goran Augustin, Mate Majerovic.
p. ; cm.
Includes bibliographical references and index.
ISBN 978-1-61122-581-5 (softcover)
1. Pregnancy--Complications. 2. Appendicitis. I. Majerovic, Mate. II. Title.
[DNLM: 1. Pregnancy Complications. 2. Abdomen, Acute. 3. Appendicitis. WQ 240]
RG580.A6A94 2010
618.3--dc22

2010037324

Published by Nova Science Publishers, Inc. † New York

Contents

Preface		vii
Chapter I	Incidence	1
Chapter II	History Taking and Clinical Examination	3
Chapter III	Examination	7
Chapter IV	Differential Diagnosis	9
Chapter V	Diagnostic Tests	11
Chapter VI	Negative Appendectomy	17
Chapter VII	Management	19
Chapter VIII	Prognosis	27
References		31
Index		41

Preface

Acute appendicitis is present in one in 500 to 2000 pregnancies (which amounts to 25% of operative indications for the acute abdomen in pregnancy). Pain in the right lower quadrant is the most reliable symptom and after the third month of pregnancy, the pain moves progressively upwards and laterally. Abdominal tenderness is almost always present and rebound tenderness in 55% to 75% patients. Fever and tachycardia may be present, but are not sensitive signs. Leukocytosis is not diagnostic as it can reach 20 x 10^9/l in early labour in normal pregnancy. A raised C reactive protein is not specific. Neutrophil granulocytosis with left shift is diagnostic of acute bacterial infection. Abdominal ultrasound is the diagnostic procedure of choice with less accuracy in the third trimester with no guidelines about the use of transvaginal ultrasound. Magnetic resonance imaging (MRI) is the diagnostic modality of choice in patients for whom the risks of radiation or the potential nephrotoxicity of iodinated contrast agents is a major concern. Multidetector row CT scan is used when there is an uncertain clinical diagnosis or equivocal laboratory or ultrasound findings, or where access to MRI is limited. Management is always surgical. This can be either by open approach (muscle splitting incision, midline vertical incision or right pararectal incision) or by laparoscopy. Fetal mortality when the appendix is not perforated is 1.5% to 5% but if perforated, it rises to 20% to 35%. Maternal mortality is less than 1%. It is rare in the first trimester, and increases with advancing gestational age and is associated with a delay in surgery of more than 24 hours and appendiceal perforation when occurs in up to 4% of patients.

Chapter I

Incidence

The first report of acute appendicitis during pregnancy was published in 1848 [1]. Acute appendicitis is the most common non-obstetric cause of acute abdomen (surgical emergency) in pregnancy. It is present in one of 500 to 2000 pregnancies and amounts to 25% of operative indications for the acute abdomen in pregnancy [2-6]. Appendicitis seems to be more common in the second trimester with incidence of 35-50% [6-8] but there are no proven data that that pregnancy affects the overall incidence of appendicitis [9]. Others claim that there is reduced incidence, especially in third trimester because of protective effect of pregnancy [10]. It is explained by suppression of TH1 mediated inflammatory response during pregnancy. Appendicitis is an inflammatory process and this observation indirectly proves that appendicitis is mediated by TH1 inflammatory response [11]. Authors comment suggest that aforementioned mechanism influence only the inflammatory causes of appendicitis but not the obstructive factor which causes gangrene due to obstruction as a secondary event. Another explanation are hormonal influences because there are incidence variations during menstrual cycle [10].

It is still not possible to presume when appendicitis would develop. Geographical differences in the incidence in appendicitis and secular trends in general population have been related to the differences and changes in the dietary intake of fibre and in standards of hygiene [12,13].

Chapter II

History Taking and Clinical Examination

The approach to pregnant patients with severe abdominal pain is similar to that for non-pregnant patients. However, the physiologic changes associated with pregnancy must be considered when interpreting findings from the history and physical examination. Thus the difficulties in diagnosis of appendicitis in pregnancy are due to:

(a) blunting of signs and symptoms due to abdominal wall distension and dislocation of intra-abdominal organs,
(b) possible changes in appendiceal location as pregnancy advances,
(c) nausea, vomiting and abdominal pain which are present in normal pregnancy especially in the first trimester.

It is important to note that there is no one reliable sign or symptom that can aid in the diagnosis of appendicitis in pregnancy, and some of the classic signs of appendicitis such as Rovsing's and psoas sign have not been shown to be of clinical significance in diagnosing an acute appendicitis in pregnancy [14].

Constant abdominal pain is the most common symptom and pain in the right lower quadrant (present in 75% of patients) is the most reliable symptom [2,3,15,16]. Classical pain migration is highly suspicious of acute appendicitis and is present in around 50% of patients [16]. After the third month of pregnancy, the pain could change location and move progressively upwards and laterally, reaching the level of the right iliac crest at the end of the sixth month of pregnancy Baer et al. [17] showed by barium enema that the growing uterus progressively displaces the appendix after the third month in a counterclockwise rotation out of the pelvis, into the upper right quadrant, by as much as two fingerbreadths above McBurney's point (Figure 1). The appendix returns to its normal position by postpartum day 10.

Others have found no evidence of upper displacement of the appendix using similar techniques [18-20]. Our opinion is that this discrepancy is probably due to the different extents of cecal fixation. In other words, a growing uterus could displace a mobile cecum with the appendix but not the completely fixed cecum. Also, due to increased separation of parietal and visceral peritoneum by an enlarging uterus there is decreased perception of somatic pain and localization, thus clinical localization of inflamed appendix is unreliable.

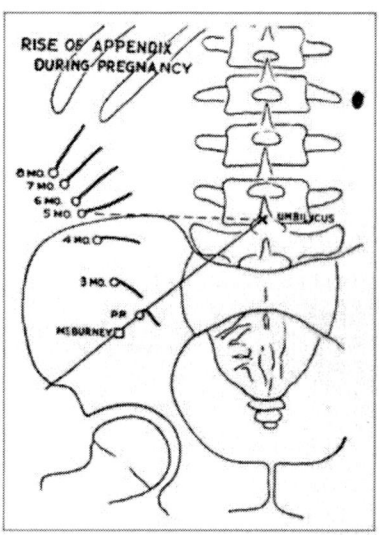

Figure 1. Change of the location of the appendix during pregnancy according to Baer et al. [17].

Nausea is nearly always present and vomiting is present in two thirds of patients. These symptoms should be evaluated with caution because many women with normal pregnancies have these symptoms especially in early pregnancy [16]. Suspicion should be raised if new-onset nausea is present (the period of nausea and vomiting in early pregnancy are mostly self-limiting and confined to the first trimester).

Anorexia is present in only one third to two thirds of pregnant patients, while it is present almost universally in nonpregnant patients [2,4,21]. If new-onset anorexia is preset it should raise suspicion, especially if present with other sings and symptoms suggesting appendicitis.

An atypical clinical picture is most commonly present in the second trimester [6]. Right upper quadrant pain, uterine contractions, dysuria, and diarrhea could also be present [8,9,14].

Chapter III

Examination

Abdominal tenderness on direct palpation is almost always present.
Rebound tenderness is present in 55% to 75% of patients [21].
Abdominal muscle rigidity is present in 50% to 65% of patients [22]. These two signs are more likely to be present during the first trimester then later in pregnancy, when laxity of the abdominal wall musculature makes this more difficult to detect.

The psoas sign is pain on passive extension of the right thigh when the inflamed appendix is in a retrocoecal/retroperitoneal location in contact with the psoas muscle. The psoas muscle is stretched by this manoeuvre. The psoas sign is observed less frequently during pregnancy when compared with non-pregnant patients with appendicitis [4].

Adler's sign is used to differentiate between appendicitis and tuboovarian pathology in RLQ pain in general population. The practitioner should find the point of maximal tenderness while the patient is supine. Then roll the patient onto left side. If pain shifts towards center then it may be tubo-ovarian. The problem in pregnant patients in third trimester is that the enlarged uterus does not allow the tubo-ovarian complex to shift its position. In study by Chen et al. [23] 36% of patients with positive appendicitis had positive Adler' sign. Unfortunately there was no comparison by trimesters of pregnancy.

The *mean maximal axillar temperature* for proven appendicitis is between 37.2-37.8°C but could be over 39°C in cases of perforation and diffuse peritonitis. Unfortunately only 50% of pregnant patients with acute appendicitis have low grade fever [24]. These temperatures are not different from normal pregnant population as is tachycardia and are not sensitive signs [8,25]. Also if normal pregnant patients have low grade fever they have leukocytosis, finding that further complicate definitive diagnosis [24]. Some studies showed an increased rate of adverse outcomes if the temperature was over 38°C [26].

Chapter IV

Differential Diagnosis

Differential diagnosis is more difficult than in nonpregnant patients because of:

(a) less reliable history and physical examination
(b) higher incidence of some pathologic conditions that mimic acute appendicitis

These conditions could be divied into nonobstetric/nongynecologic and gynecologic/obstetric conditions.

Nonobstetric/nongynecologic conditions include gastroenteritis, urinary tract infections, pyleonephritis, cholecystitis, cholelithiasis, pancreatitis, nephrolithiasis, hernia, bowel obstruction/incarcerated groin hernia, carcinoma of the large bowel, mesenteric adenitis, and rectus hematoma, pulmonary embolism, right-lower-lobe pneumonia, Meckel's diverticulitis, sickle cell disease.

Gynecologic/obstetric conditions include ruptured/hemorrhagic ovarian cyst, adnexal torsion, salpingitis, tubo-ovarian abscess, threatened abortion, placental abruption, chorioamnionitis, Pelvic inflammatory disease, degenerative fibroid, ectopic pregnancy, preeclampsia, round ligament syndrome, varicose veins in the parametria and preterm labor.

Chapter V

Diagnostic Tests

Until recently, negative appendectomy rates of 15% to 25% (and up to 50% in pregnant women) have been tolerated, given the consequences of missing a true case of appendicitis and the understanding that no test or combination of tests existed with sensitivity and specificity above 80% to 85% [26,27]. This is one of the reasons why all investigations must occur in the hospital. All the diagnostic workups should be done on an interdisciplinary basis in cooperation with the obstetrician. Physicians may be reluctant to order a radiological study because of the potential teratogenic risks to the fetus as well as the medical-legal implications of the radiation dose causing birth defects. For acute indications, the benefits for the mother usually outweigh the small risk to the fetus. The greatest effects of radiation occur during the period of rapid cell proliferation, from approximately the first week after conception through week 25. The recommended total dose of radiation during this time is less than 5 rad. During the first 2 to 3 weeks of pregnancy, while cells are not yet specialized, radiation injury will cause failure of implantation or undetectable death of the embryo. After that, injury usually occurs in the organs under development at the time of exposure. Current recommendations on radiation exposure are as follows: "No single diagnostic procedure results in a radiation dose that threatens the well-being of the developing embryo and fetus" (American College of Radiology) [28]. "Fetal risk is considered to be negligible at 5 rad or less when compared with the other risks of pregnancy, and the risk of malformations is significantly increased above control levels only at doses above 15 rad." (National Council on Radiation Protection) [29]. Exposure to less than 5 rad has not been associated with an increase in fetal anomalies or pregnancy loss" [30,31]. Also, it should be stressed that there are normal risks of pregnancy:

3% risk of spontaneous birth defects, 15% risk of spontaneous abortion, 4% risk of prematurity and growth retardation, and 1% risk of mental retardation [32]. These data should be explained to the future mother.

Laboratory Tests

Leukocytosis (raised white blood cell count – WBC) is not diagnostic as this can go up in the second and third trimesters and can reach $20 \times 10^9/l$ in early labour in normal pregnancy [33]. In view of the wide range of values, however, it is not possible to derive clinical relevance from these data [34]. For the orientation, the values over $16 \times 10^9/l$ should raise serious suspicion [3,8,22,25,26]. Unfortunately only 60% of those with perforation had values over $16 \times 10^9/l$ [16]. If there is clinical suspicion of acute appendicitis with normal values of WBC, serial WBC counts may be helpful.

Neutrophil granulocytosis with left shift: the presence of increased proportions of younger, less well differentiated neutrophils and neutrophil precursor cells in the blood is diagnostic of acute infection. If left shift is not present then granulocytosis of more than 80% should be suspicious [24].

A *raised C-reactive protein* (CRP) is not specific but with the high clinical suspicion of appendicitis it confirms the diagnosis. Some studies claim that all positive cases had negative CRP values if the patients were evaluated less than 12 h after the onset of pain [25]. Sixty-eight percent with appendicitis had CRP±10 mg/l, but all patients with perforation had elevated CRP (mean 55 mg/l) [16].

Pyuria (pus in the urine) is observed in 10% to 20% of patients with appendicitis. This may also represent concurrent asymptomatic (or symptomatic) bacteriuria found frequently in pregnant population [4]. Also mild proteinuria and/or hematuria could be present.

Transvaginal Ultrasound

There are no Royal College of Obstetricians and Gynaecologists guidelines about the use of transvaginal ultrasound. An observational study suggested that it can be used to look for the following features in acute appendicitis [35]:

The presence and size of adnexal or uterine pathology which can rule out acute appendicitis
Free fluid in the pouch of Douglas
- Abnormal pathology in the ileocoecal region; for example, appendicitis, coecal tumours, coecal diverticula, or retroperitoneal tumours.

Graded Abdominal Ultrasound

As a non-invasive procedure it is the diagnostic procedure of choice [36]. Abdominal ultrasound has good accuracy in the first and second trimesters, but has less accuracy in the third trimester. A noncompressible, blind-ended tubular structure that is visualized in the right lower quadrant with a maximal diameter greater than 6 mm is considered diagnostic. The reported sensitivity, specificity, and accuracy (overall percentage of correct test results) vary dramatically. The reported sensitivity ranges from almost 100 % [36] to only (which is by our clinical unpublished experience more precise) 40-50% [24,37]. Because its positive predictive value was 100%, it provides confirmation of the diagnosis when it is positive. However, the diagnosis of appendicitis could not be ruled out if negative. There is a significant reduction in the negative appendectomy rate in the ultrasound/CT scan group compared to clinical evaluation group or the ultrasound group. Thus, an ultrasound followed by a CT scan in patients with a normal or inconclusive ultrasound is recommended [38].

The U.S. Food and Drug Administration (FDA) has proposed an upper limit of 720 mW/cm2 for the spatial-peak temporal average intensity of the ultrasound beam for obstetric US [39]. Doppler US can produce high intensities and should be used judiciously, keeping the exposure time and acoustic output to the lowest level possible [40].

Magnetic Resonance Imaging (MRI)

Magnetic resonance imaging is the diagnostic modality of choice in patients for whom the risks of radiation or the potential nephrotoxicity of iodinated contrast agents is a major concern. It is most useful for evaluating pregnant patients with acute pain in the lower abdomen thought secondary to an extrauterine cause, such as appendicitis or ovarian torsion [41,42]. Some recommendations for its use are:

- MRI is used when the appendix is not visualised by abdominal ultrasound
- MRI is used when no other cause of an acute abdomen is found
- The patient needs to give informed consent in writing; the safety of MRI for the fetus has not been proved according to the FDA guidelines and the American College of Radiology. Thus, it is prudent to perform an MRI in pregnant patients only when ultrasound findings fail to establish a diagnosis

The significant difference between the performance of CT and MRI was not found. However, some advantages of MRI over CT include the following [43]:

- Reduced requirement for contrast administration (CT often requires rectal, oral, and/or intravenous contrast). Entire abdomen can easily be viewed in more planes.
- No radiation exposure.

MRI is not free of theoretical risks including the potential biological effects of the static and timevarying magnetic fields, the heating effects of the radiofrequency pulses, and the acoustic noise generated by the spatial encoding gradients [44]. FDA have expressed caution over the use of MRI in pregnant women and have stated that there is no conclusive evidence to establish safety [44, 45]. However, the clinical studies that have evaluated the safety of MRI during pregnancy reported no adverse effects on the developing conceptus [45]. Thus, MRI is currently preferred by radiologists over CT [46]. Thera are also some limitations and recommendations. The patient should be informed that there are no known harmful effects from use of MR imaging at 1.5 T or lower magnetic field strengths [47] and that there is lack of experience with use of field strengths greater than 2.5 T, and they should be avoided at present [48]. Also absolute contraindication for MR are metal implants in the body that are not made of titanium or the composition is not known.

Computed Tomography (CT) Scan

In 1998, Rao et al. published their experience with the use of a helical or spiral CT technique and results show that the method is highly sensitive and specific for the identification of acute appendicitis in the nonobstetric population with lower costs when CT scanning was used to diagnose appendicitis with sensitivity, specificity, and diagnostic accuracy each of 98%. [49,50]. Appendix CT scans were identified as positive for appendicitis on the basis of an enlarged appendix (>6 mm in the maximum diameter) and periappendiceal inflammatory changes, such as fat stranding, phlegmon, fluid collection, and extraluminal gas. Unfortunately, there are instances where the findings at CT scan are not so clear. Several authors comment on "equivocal" readings. In all instances, the "equivocal" readings influence on the sensitivity and specificity of CT scan, depending on how these readings were handled.

It is preferable to use the multidetector row CT scan with high speed mode in pregnant patients since it has half the radiation dose of the high quality mode and its scanning parameters are otherwise identical. Radiation exposure using this test is 300 mrad, which is below an accepted safe level of radiation exposure in pregnancy of 5 rad. Sensitivity and specificity in a pregnant population with acute appendicitis are similar to general population with values reaching 100% [51]. Limitations include small number of patients (seven), retrospective study and study performed in a tertiary care institution, therefore these findings may not be universally applicable. In a letter to the editor in response to that series, CT scan was not helpful in the diagnosis in a single patient. Authors comments on the aforementioned study included the advanced appendicitis with periappendicitis and laparotomy with a paramedian incision. Indirectly this meant that the 100% sensitivity and specificity was because of significant pathologic changes in advanced appendicitis [52].

The conclusion and recommendation is that the CT scan should be used when there is an uncertain clinical diagnosis or equivocal laboratory or ultrasound findings, or where access to MRI is limited.

Chest Radiograph

It may be useful in identifying right lower lobe pneumonia from appendicitis in pregnant patients with right-sided abdominal pain. A plain abdominal radiograph can be used to identify air fluid levels or free air but indicated according to signs and symptoms of perforation (sudden sharp and severe pain...) or obstruction (significant or feculent vomiting, no stool and flatus evacuation for several days).

Diagnostic Algorithm

Diagnostic algorithm is presented on Figure 2.

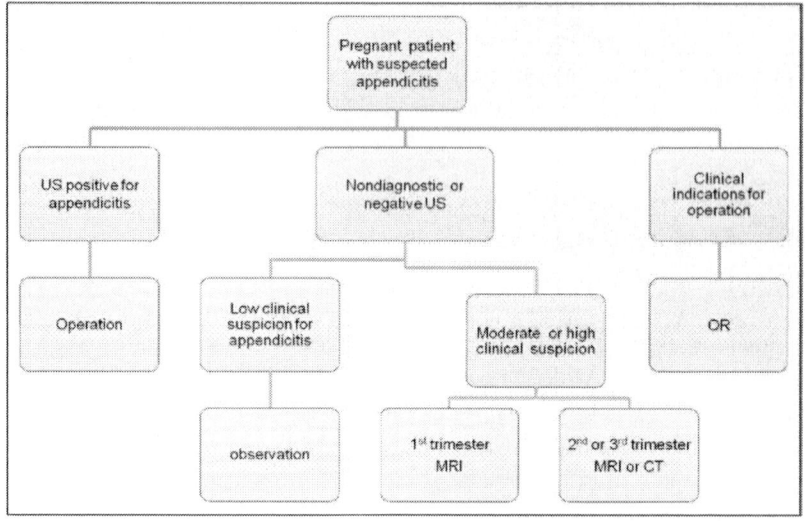

Figure 2. Algorithm for the evaluation of pregnant patients with suspected appendicitis [53].

Chapter VI

Negative Appendectomy

There is still a dilemma to perform or not a laparoscopic appendectomy if the appendix looks macroscopically normal in the non-pregnant patient, as well as among the population with no other abdominopelvic pathology. It has been argued that retaining a normal-looking appendix allows it to be used in reconstructive procedures [54]. On the other hand, some investigators believe that the appendix should be removed to rule out appendicitis histologically, also making the diagnosis of appendicitis less likely if the patient's symptoms return [55]. It can partly be explained by the fact that gross changes are not visible if intramural, mucosal and submucosal changes in appendix are present histologically and could be responsible for the symptoms. Van den Broek et al. reported that 9% of their series continued to have recurrent RLQ pain after negative laparoscopy, yet they did not recommend appendectomy in these patients [56]. This is due to early intraluminal inflammation that subsequently leads to transmural inflammation or the inflammation subsides and could lead to chronic appendicitis with recurrent episodes of right lower quadrant pain and other symptoms mimicking acute appendicitis. Several studies report 20-22% of patients with clinical suspicion of acute appendicitis who underwent appendectomy, responded very well to appendectomy in spite of a normal microscopical examination of the appendix. Explanation could be found in other underlying causes such as appendix colic, appendicular feacolith and functional appendicular abnormality or functional appendicopathy that might be the contributory factors rather than acute inflammation [57,58]. In recent study of laparoscopic appendectomy there were 30% of intraoperative diagnosis of normal appendix confirmed inflammed histologicaly. Authors recommend appendectomy in these situations [59]. These conclusions are similar to SAGES guidelines for laparoscopic appendectomy (04 / 2009): *If no other pathology is identified, the decision to remove the appendix should be considered but based on the individual clinical scenario (level III, Grade A). Macroscopically normal appendixes may have abnormal histopathology. Several studies have shown a 19% to 40% rate of pathologically abnormal appendix in the setting of no visual abnormalities. Therefore the risk of leaving a potentially abnormal appendix must be weighed against the risk of appendectomy in each individual scenario.*

Furthermore, some neoplasms of the appendix can occur in an organ that appears grossly unremarkable [60,61]. If pseudomyxoma peritonei is observed, the appendix should always be removed and subjected to thorough histologic examination.

Conclusion in one sentence should be: As a surgeon you should not be deterred from removing an appendix once the diagnosis is suspected, because pregnancy is not affected by removal of a normal appendix [62].

Chapter VII

Management

Once investigations have been carried out in hospital and the diagnosis of acute appendicitis has been confirmed, management is always surgical removal of the inflamed appendix. This can be performed by several different procedures simply divided into laparotomy or laparoscopy procedures.

Anesthetic Considerations in the Pregnant Patient

Anesthetic concerns in the pregnant patient can be broken down into two major categories: teratogenicity of the anesthetic agents and maternal physiologic changes as a result of anesthetic agents. The teratogenicity of anesthetic agents, defined as the potential effect in chromosomal damage or in carcinogenesis in the fetus, is minimal [63]. In a consensus statement printed in the *New England Journal of Medicine* in 2000, no anesthetic agents were listed as definitively causative of fetal malformations [64]. Increased oxygen consumption and mechanical displacement of the abdominal organs cause the pregnant patient to increase minute ventilation, primarily through a 30% to 40% increase in tidal volume [65]. A compensatory respiratory alkalosis with a PaCO2 from 30 to 35 mm Hg develops. Intubation may be more difficult because of increased airway edema later in the pregnancy, and smaller endotracheal tubes should be used at this time. Because decreased lower esophageal sphincter pressure and delayed gastric emptying in pregnancy can cause an increased risk of aspiration, cricoid pressure should be used to prevent aspiration during intubation [66]. End-tidal CO_2 monitoring should be used intraoperatively. Hypotension in the pregnant patient should be treated initially with aggressive intravenous fluid resuscitation. The patient should be placed in the left lateral decubitus position, if possible, to increase venous return. Trendelenburg positioning can also be used in the hypotensive patient to increase venous return [63].

Open Appendectomy

As in other surgical procedures type of incision is very important for successful completion of the operation. Despite the type of incision used the operation should be completed with minimal uterine manipulation. There are several incisions that could be performed. Despite the surgical approach, the most experienced abdominal surgeon should perform the procedure to shorten the operation time and possible postoperative complications as much as possible.

Muscle Splitting Incision (Mcburney's Incision, Gridiron Incision)

This is the incision of choice for open approach for the removal of the appendix in pregnant patients in all trimesters. In the latter pregnancy the incision could be positioned above McBurney's incision because of possible displacement of the appendix in the right upper quadrant. This change of the location of the incision is not necessary because the appendix was easily located in 94% of the incisions made through McBurney's point and in 80% of the incisions made above McBurney's point [67].

Midline Vertical Incision

This incision is used when acute abdomen with diffuse peritoneal irritation is present. This is important for two main reasons:

1) it allows the surgeon to deal with unexpected surgical findings
2) it allows caesarean delivery if necessary

Right Transrectal of Pararectal Incision

These incisions are rarely used. If the diagnosis is certain than McBurney's incision is made. If acute abdomen with diffuse peritoneal irritation is present than midline vertical incision is made.

Laparoscopic Appendectomy

Laparoscopic appendectomy during pregnancy continues to be controversial especially in latter second and third trimester. Several case reports and small series have reported success during all trimesters without complications [26,68,69] but in the same institutions there is higer percentage of open approach during the third trimester [26]. Thus there is some bias in these studies and conclusions are not yet presented as recommendations.

In the case of appendicitis, some might argue that the laparoscopic approach exposes the fetus to excessive risks from trocar placement and the effects of carbon dioxide on the developing fetus and the long-term effects of this exposure with significant fetal loss [70,71]. Laparoscopic procedures are approximately 50% longer with conflicting studies showing decreased length of stay and hospitalization [72,73] but with increasing number of laparoscopic procedures performed worldwide the duration of open and laparoscopic operations would become the same [26]. Questions arise regarding the risk for decreased uterine blood flow due to increased intra-abdominal pressures from insufflation and the possibility of fetal carbon dioxide absorption [74]. Carbon dioxide used for the creation of pneumoperitoneum could lead to fetal carbon dioxide absorption with potential subsequent fetal acidosis. This could be minimized with maintenance of intra-abdominal pressure <12 mm Hg and minimizing operative time. Clinical and experimental studies found no substantial adverse effects for the fetus when the maximal pneumoperitoneum pressure was limited to 10 to 12 mmHg and a duration of less then 60 minutes [75,76]. Others stress the importance of the absorption of carbon monoxide, produced by the use of monopolar energy, through the peritoneum. The absorbed carbon monoxide can produce carboxyhemoglobin and metahemoglobin that compete with hemoglobin in the uptake and transport of oxygen. It is recommended to continually remove the smoke produced by tissue fulguration [77]. Harmonic scissors produce vapor-free gas, avoiding the potential effects of carbon monoxide [78]. Other negative effect of electrocautery is the potential for uterine irritation.

There are many advantages of laparoscopic technique. Authors note that laparoscopy expands the ability to explore the abdomen with less uterine manipulation [79]. Further, it increases the ability to locate and treat the ectopic appendix and results in relatively small incisions compared with the open technique or helps in detecting other unexpected sources of pain [80,81]. With open technique of trocar placement there is almost no possibility of injury of intra-abdominal organs. Direct uterine injury during trocar placement has been reported but without fetal loss [82]. Also reduced cecal manipulation during appendectomy with less cecal trauma causes earlier restore of large bowel function, earlier passage of the first flatus and first postoperative stool (authors clinical observation, not published results). In addition to general advantage of a smaller incisions, less postoperative pain, and earlier return to normal activity, laparoscopy can result in less manipulation of the uterus while obtaining optimum exposure of the surgical field. Lower rates of dehiscence or herniation during labor are another potential benefit. Rapid return to full activity could reduce the frequency of maternal thrombosis and embolic events, which can be a source of maternal mortality in some patients and it is known that thromboembolic events are more common in prengancy [75,81,83]. Some studies found significantly shorter hospital stay in the laparoscopic group (3.4 vs. 4.2 days) [26]. A study from the Swedish Health Registry evaluated 2,233 laparoscopic and 2,491 open laparotomy cases from 2 million deliveries in Sweden from 1973 to 1993 [84]. Outcomes evaluated birth weight, gestational duration, intrauterine growth retardation, congenital malformations, stillbirths, and neonatal deaths with no statistically significant differences comparing the laparoscopy and laparotomy group. It appears that there was an increased risk for infants in both laparoscopy and laparotomy groups to weigh less than 2,500 g, to be delivered before 37 weeks, and to have an increased incidence of growth restriction compared with the total population.

Current Practical/Clincal SAGES guidelines (04 / 2009) statement is: *Laparoscopic appendectomy may be performed safely in pregnant patients with suspicion of appendicitis (Level II, Grade B). Laparoscopic appendectomy can be performed safely in any trimester and is considered by* many to be the standard of care for gravid patients with suspected appendicitis.

Laparoscopic Technique

In the first and early second trimester the technique is similar as in non-pregnant patients. In an advanced pregnancy the port positions are somewhat specific (see further text). The patient is placed supine on the operating room table. Restraining straps are placed across the chest and thighs and sequential pneumatic compression devices are places on both lower extremities. A Foley catheter and a nasogastric tube are placed and removed at the end of the operation. A prophylactic antibiotic is administered intravenously 30 minutes before the skin incision. Maternal end-tidal CO_2 is monitored and should be controlled within physiologic range (30 to 40 mm Hg).

Patients are tilted to the left to displace the uterus from the IVC and to remove the small bowel from the operating field and a slight Trendelenburg position may be added, if necessary. The procedure is always performed using 3 ports, and their placement is modified in accordance with gestational age. In the advanced pregnancy the first port (5 or 10 mm - laparoscope) is placed 2-4 cm cephalad to the gravid uterus in the upper midline between the umbilicus and xiphoid process. The bigger the uterus the more cranial the first trocar is placed for easier intraperitoneal manipulation.

Pneumoperitoneum is carried out using an open (Hasson) technique for entering the abdominal cavity under direct vision. Other possibility is to use a Veress needle but with the higher risk of perforation of intra-abdominal organs or pneumoamnion [85,86]. Also an optical trocar can be used for entering the abdomen. The pneumoperitoneum pressure is maintained between 10-12mm Hg. The second port (5 or 12 mm) is placed laterally in the right lower quadrant, and the third port (5 or 10 mm) is placed in the right upper quadrant in a more cranial location. There are several modifications of instrument placement and their size depending on the laparoscopic tehcnique and equipment. Twelve mm ports are used when the linear cutting stapler is used for the transection of the appendix at its base. Fetal heart rate is recorded immediately before and after surgery and during operation in the lower left quadrant without desufflation. (Figure 3).

All the extracted specimens should be sent to patohistological examination because in this pregnant patient group other pathologies other than appendicitis (including carcinoid tumor) could be found [26].

Nasogastric tube is extracted after the operation. Oral intake is started on the first postoperative day.

Conversion from Laparoscopic to Open Approach

The question could arise about influence of conversion from laparoscopic to open approach to mother and fetus. Studies did not show increased rate of complications and increased maternal or fetal mortality and preterm delivery. In the open approach group preterm delivery rate was 11.8% versus 15.8% in the laparoscopic approach [87]. Caution should be present because of a small number of patients that had underwent such conversions [87]. Theoretically if conversion is indicated then mostly: 1) the anatomy is difficult or 2) inflammation is in an advanced stage in the form of perforation or abscess. Both situations are connected to longer operative time and higher percentage of complications.

Risk of Drug-Induced Congenital Defects

There are many categories of drugs that could have deleterious effects on a fetus and the detailed elaboration is out of the scope of this book. There are two main categories of medications used in all patients either prophylactically or therapeutically. All teratogenic drugs generally determine a specific pattern or single malformation during a sensitive period of gestation with a dose-dependent effect [88].

Antibiotics should be administered preoperatively (30-60 min prior to skin incision) in all patients (administered to 94% of patients found in the literature) [72]. These should be from the FDA class B drugs which are found to be safe for the fetus. Standard antibiotics in use are second-generation cephalosporins which comprise 60% of all classes of antibiotics used during pregnancy for acute appendicitis found in literature [72]. If a gangrenous or perforated appendix is found cephalosporins are used in combination with metronidazole (FDA class B) [14].

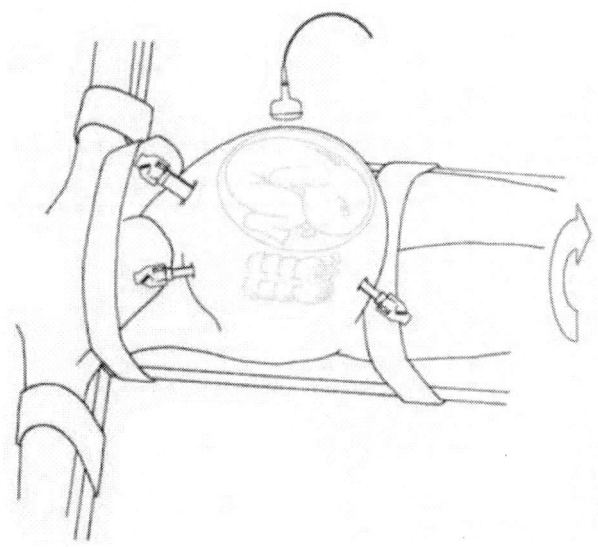

Figure 3. Patient positioning, port placement and intraoperative fetal monitoring for laparoscopic appendectomy in advanced pregnancy (see text for details) [89].

Use of NSADs during the second and third trimesters is associated with oligohydramnios and anuria and, close to term, to precocious closure of Botalli's duct, with subsequent pulmonary hypertension, intracranial haemorrhage and necrotising enterocolitis (NEC) [90-95]. During pregnancy the drug of choice for analgesic, anti-inflammatory and antipyretic action is paracetamol. When appendectomy is performed with Cesarean section through median laparotomy then all classes of medications could be used as in non-pregnant patients unless contraindicated for maternal reasons.

Incidental Meckel's Diverticulum (MD) During Exploration

Symptomatic MD during pregnancy is exceptionally rare. Walser et al. in 1962 published the first report of Meckel's diverticulitis in a pregnant woman [96]. Only 23 cases of MD complicating pregnancy have been reported up to date [97]. In the pregnant patient, the average maternal age of all reported cases of symptomatic MD was 24 years (14-31 years). The most common complication was perforation (57%), maternal mortality was 16%, fetal mortality was 13%, and the incidence of preterm deliveries was 25%

[97]. Given the high incidence of perforation resulting in an enormous rate of maternal and fetal mortality, removal of incidentally found MD is justified in the pregnant patient [97]. An epidemiologic, population-based study from the Mayo Clinic demonstrates that the benefits from removal of an incidental MD in general population are far superior than the risk of developing complications. Authors found that if the patient fulfill any of the following criteria (or combination):

(1) patient age younger than 50 years
(2) male sex
(3) MD length greater than 2 cm
(4) ectopic or abnormal features within a diverticulum

then there is an indication for the incidental MD to be removed. Their data show that when 1 criterion is met, the overall proportion of symptomatic MD was 17%. When 2, 3, or all 4 criteria were met, the proportion increased to 25%, 42%, and 70%, respectively [98].

During open approach, if the asimptomatic MD or symptomatic Meckel's diverticulitis is found, *diverticulectomy* or *wedge small bowel resection* with subsequent bowel continuity is peformed. Laparoscopic surgical technique is the same as in non-pregnant population. An endoscopic linear cutting stapler is introduced through a 12-mm trocar and applied to the base of the MD, perpendicular to the base of the MD but transverse to the longitudinal axis of the bowel. The stapler is fired and the MD resected off the ileum. Small bleeding points at the edge of the staple line, if present, are sutured intracorporeally with 3-0 Vicryl. All the specimens are delivered through 12-mm port with the use of an endobag. A wedge resection is not necessary in these incidental findings because the base of the MD is not inflamed. If necessary endoscopic linear cutting staplers are used for the excision, and bowel continuity achieved by placing intracorporeal sutures with 2-0 Vicryl. Pathologic specimen should always be sent for pathohistologic examination.

Chapter VIII

Prognosis

Perforation Rate

Perforation rates for pregnant patients have been reported as high as 55% compared to 4-19% of the general population [72,99]. Delay in diagnosis leads to appendiceal perforation. As in non-pregnant patients it has many potential deleterious consequences. In cases of pregnant patients these consequences imply to both mother and fetus. Trend in overall perforation rate is lowering from 25% [100] to 15% during last 2 decades [6]. The rate of perforation through the trimesters is increasing 8.7%, 12.5% and 26.1%, respectively [6]. A 66% perforation rate has been reported when operation is delayed by more than 24 hours compared with 0% incidence when surgical management is initiated prior to 24 hours after presentation [99]. This is one of the most important observations for the surgeons and gynecologists. There are several causes for the treatment delay [101]:

(a) atypical clinical picture with uncertain diagnosis when watchful waiting is indicated
(b) significant time consumption during consultations between the gynecologist and surgeon if institutions are dislocated
(c) time consumption during the transfer of the patient when the departments and institutions are dislocated

The difficulty in making a clinical diagnosis particularly close to term combined with the previously quoted high incidences of fetal and maternal mortality for appendiceal perforation has led to a traditionally low threshold for surgical intervention. This is partly due to inacurate preoperative diagnostic imaging. This has resulted in a higher negative appendectomy rate, ranging from 23% to 55% in pregnant women compared with 18% in nonpregnant women [8,10,83,102-105]. The first trimester yields a greater accuracy, but more than 40% of patients in the second and third trimester will have a normal appendix [106]. Perforation can also result in an increased risk of generalized peritonitis because the omentum cannot isolate the infection [9, 107].

Fetal Mortality

Appendicitis is the most common surgical cause of fetal loss during pregnancy because of its frequency during pregnancy and frequently atypical clinical picture with delayed diagnosis and treatment [108]. In 1908, Babler reported more than 200 cases of appendicitis in pregnancy with maternal mortality of 24% and a fetal mortality of 40%. As a result of this review, Babler claimed that *the mortality of appendicitis complicating pregnancy is the mortality of delay* [109]. Today the combined miscarriage/fetal mortality when the appendix is not perforated is 1.5-5% [6,15,24,110,111]. When the appendix is perforated, fetal mortality raises to 20-36% [6,14,24,102,110,112,113]. It should be stated that the data presented in many articles have included retrospective studies for the collection of sufficient number of patients for data analysis using extended time periods. In many of these articles fetal mortality was higher in years before 1990 at a time when the current possibilities offered by modern neonatology, fast and accurate diagnostic workup, intensive care and antibiotic therapy were limited or not available.

The problem raised in some articles was the rate of fetal loss of 3% after negative laparotomy and appendectomy of normal appendix. Some of these investigators included complications in long-term follow-up after appendectomy and did not take into account the expected number of perinatal and intrauterine deaths in the total (normal) pregnant population [62,99]. A similar observation was found by McGory et al. and there was one topic that should be discussed further. It should be noted that in 15% of negative appendectomies another pathology was found. Mostly these pathologic findings were of genital origin and in this subgroup of patients with the diagnosis of leiomyoma or inflammation of the uterus there was significantly higher incidence of fetal loss and early delivery [104]. Others concluded that if there was an effect of surgical trauma on the feto-placentaruterine elements it should, in uncomplicated cases, have ceased approximately 1 week after appendectomy. This increased risk of delivery the week following surgery was present when performed after 23 weeks' gestation [8]. Any complication and increased risk of preterm delivery after that period in a patient without surgical complications should not be related to the operation itself [102,111].

Premature delivery rate was often omitted in reports on appendicitis, but it ranges between 15% and 45% [3,114,115]. Different agents have been used as tocolytic agents prophylactically like magnesium sulphate, terbutaline or 17-hydroxyprogesterone [116,117]. Beta2-receptor agonist (Ritodrine) is perhaps the most used tocolytic agent. Some authors claim that tocolytic treatment after the onset of contractions could not prevent preterm labor and should be ordered for the patients with delayed presentation and advanced gestational age in order to prevent preterm labor and fetal loss [37]. No study has documented positive effects on outcome. The current conclusion and recommendation is that the use of these agents are a matter of choice. [102,116,118].

Maternal Mortality

Overall, maternal mortality is less than 1% [9,14,16,102]. It is rare in the first trimester, and increases with advancing gestational age [62]. It is associated with:

- A delay in surgery of more than 24 hours after onset of symptoms [3,99]
- Appendiceal perforation (when maternal mortality occurs in up to 4% of patients) [100,113]

The risk of perforation increases with gestational age, and perforation in the third trimester often results in preterm labor [9]. The risk for premature delivery is the greatest during the first week after surgery. Others find similar risk factors for adverse outcome and also included: maternal temperature greater than 38°C, leukocytosis greater than $16 \times 10^9/l$, or more than 48 h between onset of symptoms and emergency room presentation [26].

References

[1] Hancock H. Disease of the appendix caeci cured by operation. *Lancet.* 1848;ii:380-382.

[2] Gomez A, Wood M. Acute appendicitis during pregnancy. *Am. J. Surg.* 1979;137:180-3.

[3] Horowitz MD, Gomez GA, Santiesteban R, Burkett G. Acute appendicitis during pregnancy. Diagnosis and management. *Arch. Surg.* 1985;120:1362-7.

[4] Bailey LE, Finley RK Jr, Miller SF, Jones LM. Acute appendicitis during pregnancy. *Am. Surg.* 1986; 52: 218-21.

[5] Sivanesaratnam V. The acute abdomen and the obstetrician. *Baillieres Best Pract. Res. Clin. Obstet. Gynaecol.* 2000; 14: 89-102.

[6] Ueberrueck T, Koch A, Meyer L, Hinkel M, Gastinger I. Ninety-four appendectomies for suspected acute appendicitis during pregnancy. *World J. Surg.* 2004;28:508-11

[7] Kazim SF, Pal KM. Appendicitis in pregnancy: experience of thirty-eight patients diagnosed and managed at a tertiary care hospital in Karachi. *Int. J. Surg.* 2009;7:365-7.

[8] Mourad J, Elliott JP, Erickson L, Lisboa L. Appendicitis in pregnancy: new information that contradicts long-held clinical beliefs. *Am. J. Obstet. Gynecol.* 2000; 182: 1027-9.

[9] Tracey M, Fletcher HS. Appendicitis in pregnancy. *Am. Surg.* 2000;66:555–560.

[10] Andersson RE, Lambe M. Incidence of appendicitis during pregnancy. *Int. J. Epidemiol.* 2001;30:1281-5.

[11] Confavreux C, Hutchingson M, Hours MM et al. Rate of pregnancy-related relapses in multiple sclerosis. *N. Engl. J. Med.* 1998;339:285-91.

[12] Burkitt DP. Aetiology of the appendicitis *Br. J. Surg.* 1971;58:695-99.

[13] Barker DJP. Acute appendicitis and dietary fibre: an alternative hypothesis. *Br. Med. J.* 1985;290:1125-27.
[14] Al-Mulhim AA. Acute appendicitis in pregnancy. A review of 52 cases. *Int. Surg.* 1996;81:295–7.
[15] Babaknia A, Parsa H, Woodruff JD. Appendicitis during pregnancy. *Obstet. Gynecol.* 1977;50:40-4.
[16] Andersen B, Nielsen TF. Appendicitis in pregnancy: diagnosis, management and complications. *Acta Obstet. Gynecol. Scand.* 1999;78:758-62.
[17] Baer JL, Reis RA, Arens RA. Appendicitis in pregnancy: with changes in position and axis of the normal appendix in pregnancy. *JAMA.* 1932;98:1359–64.
[18] Fink K. Monatschr, f Gerburtsch. *U. Gynak.* 1925;71:328.
[19] Hoffmann K. *Arch. f. Gynak.* 1920;112:230.
[20] Hodjati H, Kazerooni T. Location of the appendix in the gravid patient: a re-evaluation of the established concept. *Int. J. Gynaecol. Obstet.* 2003;81:245–7.
[21] Richards C, Daya S. Diagnosis of acute appendicitis in pregnancy. *Can. J. Surg.* 1989;32:358-60.
[22] Cunningham FG, McCubbin JH. Appendicitis complicating pregnancy. *Obstet. Gynecol.* 1975;45:415–20.
[23] Chen CF, Yen SJ, Tan KH et al. Acute appendicitis during pregnancy. *J. Med. Sci.* 1999;19:256-262.
[24] Zhang Y, Zhao YY, Qiao J, Ye RH. Diagnosis of appendicitis during pregnancy and perinatal outcome in the late pregnancy. *Chin. Med. J. (Engl).* 2009;122:521-4.
[25] Hoshino T, Ihara Y, Suzuki T. Appendicitis during pregnancy. *Int. J. Gynaecol. Obstet.* 2000;69:271-3.
[26] Sadot E, Telem DA, Arora M, Butala P, Nguyen SQ, Divino CM. Laparoscopy: a safe approach to appendicitis during pregnancy. *Surg. Endosc.* 2010;24:383-9.
[27] Flum DR, Morris A, Koespell T, Dellinger EP. Has misdiagnosis of appendicitis decreased over time? A population-based analysis. *JAMA.* 2001;286:1748–53.
[28] Hall EJ. Scientific view of low level radiation risks. *Radiographics.* 1991;11:509–18.
[29] National Council on Radiation Protection and Measurements. Medical radiation exposure of pregnant and potentiall pregnant women. NCRP report no. 54. Bethesda, MD: NCRP, 1977.

[30] American College of Obstetrics and Gynecology, ACOG, Committee on Obstetric Practice. Guidelines for diagnostic imaging during pregnancy. ACOG Committee opinion no. 299., 2004.
[31] Subramaniam R, Amorosa JK. Imaging the pregnant patient for nonobstetric conditions: algorithms and radiation dose considerations. *Radiographics.* 2007;27:1705-22.
[32] Brent RL, Mettler FA. Pregnancy policy. *AJR Am. J. Roentgenol.* 2004;182:819–822.
[33] Amos JD, Schorr SJ, Norman PF, et al. Laparoscopic surgery during pregnancy. *Am. J. Surg.* 1997;174:222.
[34] Viktrup L, Hee P. Appendicitis during pregnancy. *Am. J. Obstet. Gynecol.* 2001;185:259–260.
[35] Caspi B, Zbar AP, Mavor E, et al. The contribution of transvaginal ultrasound in the diagnosis of acute appendicitis: an observational study. *Ultrasound Obstet. Gynecol.* 2003;21:273-6.
[36] Lim HK, Bae SH, Seo GS. Diagnosis of acute appendicitis in pregnant women: value of sonography. *AJR.* 1992;159:539–42.
[37] Yilmaz HG, Akgun Y, Bac B, et al. Acute appendicitis in pregnancy–risk factors associated with principal outcomes: a case control study. *Int. J. Surg.* 2007;5:192–197.
[38] Wallace CA, Petrov MS, Soybel DI, Ferzoco SJ, Ashley SW, Tavakkolizadeh A. Influence of imaging on the negative appendectomy rate in pregnancy. *J. Gastrointest. Surg.* 2008;12:46-50.
[39] Barnett SB. Routine ultrasound scanning in first trimester: what are the risks? *Semin. Ultrasound CT MR.* 2002;23:387–391.
[40] Abramowicz JS, Kossoff G, Marsal K, Ter Haar G. Safety Statement, 2000 (reconfirmed 2003). International Society of Ultrasound in Obstetrics and Gynecology (ISUOG). *Ultrasound Obstet. Gynecol.* 2003;21:100.
[41] Kanal E, Borgstede JP, Barkovich AJ, et al. American College of Radiology White Paper on MR Safety: 2004 update and revisions. *AJR Am. J. Roentgenol.* 2004;182:1111– 4.
[42] Singh A, Danrad R, Hahn PF, et al. MR imaging of the acute abdomen and pelvis: acute appendicitis and beyond. *Radiographics.* 2007;27:1419-31.
[43] Cobben LP, Groot I, Haans L, et al. MRI for clinically suspected appendicitis during pregnancy. *AJR Am. J. Roentgenol.* 2004;183:671–675.

[44] De Wilde JP, Rivers AW, Price DL. A review of the current use of magnetic resonance imaging in pregnancy and safety implications for the fetus. *Prog. Biophys. Mol. Biol.* 2005;87:335–353.
[45] Chen MM, Coakley FV, Kaimal A, et al. Guidelines for computed tomography and magnetic resonance imaging use during pregnancy and lactation. *Obstet. Gynecol.* 2008;112(2 pt 1):333–340.
[46] Brown MA. Imaging acute appendicitis. Seminin Ultrasound CT MR 2008;29:293–307.
[47] Shellock FG, Crues JV. MR procedures: biologic effects, safety, and patient care. *Radiology.* 2004;232:635–652.
[48] Wagner LK, Lester RG, Saldana LR. Exposure of the pregnant patient to diagnostic radiations: a guide to medical management. 2nd ed. Madison, Wis: Medical Physics, 1997.
[49] Rao PM, Rhea JT, Novelline RA, Mostafavi AA, McCabe CJ. Effect of computed tomography of the appendix on treatment of patients and use of hospital resources. *N. Engl. J. Med.* 1998;338:141–6.
[50] Rao P, Rhea J, Novelline R, McCabe C, Lawrason J, Berger D, et al. Helical CT technique for the diagnosis of appendicitis: prospective evaluation of a focused appendix CT examination. *Radiology.* 1997;202:139-44.
[51] Ames Castro M, Shipp TD, Castro EE, Ouzounian J, Rao P. The use of helical computed tomography in pregnancy for the diagnosis of acute appendicitis. *Am. J. Obstet. Gynecol.* 2001;184:954-7.
[52] Dupuis O, Audra P, Mellier G. Is helical computed tomography 100% sensitive to diagnose acute appendicitis during pregnancy? *Am. J. Obstet. Gynecol.* 2002;186:336
[53] Freeland M, King E, Safcsak K, Durham R. Diagnosis of appendicitis in pregnancy. *Am. J. Surg.* 2009;198:753-8
[54] Wheeler Ra, Malone PS: Use of the appendix in reconstructive surgery. A case against incidental appendectomy. *Br. J. Surg.* 1991;78:1283-1285.
[55] Wilcox RT, Traverse LW: Have the evaluation and treatment of acute appendicitis changed with new technology? *Surg. Clin. North Am.* 1997;77:1355-1370.
[56] van den Broek WT, Bijnen AB, de Ruiter P, Gouma DJ. A normal appendix found during diagnostic laparoscopy should not be removed. *Br. J. Surg.* 2001; 88:251-4.
[57] Hussain A, Mahmood H, Singhal T, Balakrishnan S, El-Hasani S. What is positive appendicitis? A new answer to an old question.

Clinical, macroscopical and microscopical findings in 200 consecutive appendectomies. *Singapore Med. J.* 2009;50:1145-9.

[58] Wang Y, Reen DJ, Puri P. Is a histologically normal appendix following emergency appendicectomy always normal. *Lancet.* 1996; 347:1076-9.

[59] Phillips AW, Jones AE, Sargen K. Should the macroscopically normal appendix be removed during laparoscopy for acute right iliac fossa pain when no other explanatory pathology is found? *Surg. Laparosc. Endosc. Percutan Tech.* 2009;19:392-4.

[60] Carr NJ, McCarthy WF, Sobin LH Epithelial noncarcinoid tumors and tumor-like lesions of the appendix: A clinicopathologic study of 184 patientswith a multivariate analysis ofprognostic factors. *Cancer.* 1995;75:757-768.

[61] Carr NJ, Sobin LH: Unusual tumors of the appendix and pseudomyxoma peritonei. *Semin. Diagn. Pathol.* 1996;13:314-325.

[62] Halvorsen AC, Brandt B, Andreasen JJ. Acute appendicitis in pregnancy: complications and subsequent management. *Eur. J. Surg.* 1992;158:603–6.

[63] Melnick DM, Wahl WL, Dalton VK. Management of general surgical problems in the pregnant patient. *Am. J. Surg.* 2004;187:170-80.

[64] Gideon Koren G, Pastuszak A, Ito S. Drugs in pregnancy. *N. Engl. J. Med.* 1998;338:1128–37.

[65] Gordon MC. Maternal physiology in pregnancy. In: Gabbe SG, Niebyl JR, Simpson JL, editors. Obstetrics: normal and problem pregnancies. 4th ed. New York: Churchill Livingstone, 2002, p 63–91.

[66] Pedersen H, Finster M. Anesthetic risk in the pregnant surgical patient. *Anesthesiology.* 1979;51:439–51.

[67] Popkin CA, Lopez PP, Cohn SM, Brown M, Lynn M. The incision of choice for pregnant women with appendicitis is through McBurney's point. *Am. J. Surg.* 2002;183:20-2.

[68] Schreiber JH. Laparoscopic appendectomy in pregnancy. *Surg. Endosc.* 1990;4:100–102.

[69] Gurbuz AT, Peetz ME. The acute abdomen in the pregnant patient. *Surg. Endosc.* 1997;11:98–102.

[70] Rizzo AG. Laparoscopic surgery in pregnancy: longterm follow-up. *J. Laparoendosc. Adv. Surg. Tech. A.* 2003;13:11–15.

[71] Amos D, Schorr SJ, Norman PF, et al. Laparoscopic surgery during pregnancy. *Am. J. Surg.* 1996;171:435–438.

[72] Hale DA, Molloy M, Pearl RH, et al. Appendectomy: a contemporary appraisal. *Ann. Surg.* 1997;225:252–61.
[73] Lachman E, Schienfeld A, Voss E, et al. Pregnancy and laparoscopic surgery. *J. Am. Assoc. Gynecol. Laparosc.* 1999;6:347–51.
[74] Sharp HT. The acute abdomen during pregnancy. *Clin. Obstet. Gynecol.* 2002;45:405–13.
[75] Curet MJ. Special problems in laparoscopic surgery. Previous abdominal surgery, obesity, and pregnancy. *Surg. Clin. North Am.* 2000;80:1093–1110.
[76] Curet MJ, Vogt DA, Schob O, et al. Effects of CO_2 pneumoperitoneum in pregnant ewes. *J. Surg. Res.* 1996;63:339–344.
[77] Beebe DS, Swica H, Carlson N, et al. High levels of carbon monoxide are produced by electro-cautery of tissue during laparoscopic cholecystectomy. *Anesth. Anal.* 1993;77:338–341.
[78] Barrett WL, Garber SM. Surgical smoke—a review of the literature. Is this just a lot of hot air? *Surg. Endosc.* 2003;17:979–987.
[79] Bennett TL, Estes N. Laparoscopic cholecystectomy in the second trimester of pregnancy: a case report. *J. Reprod. Med.* 1993;38:833–834.
[80] Lyass S, Pikarsky A, Eisenberg VH, Elchalal U, Schenker JG, Reissman P. Is laparoscopic appendicectomy safe in pregnant women? *Surg. Endosc.* 2001;15:377–379.
[81] de Perrot MD, Jenny A, Morales M, Kohlik M, Morel P. Laparoscopic appendicectomy during pregnancy. *Surg. Laparosc. Endosc. Percutan Tech.* 2000;10:368–371.
[82] Reedy MB, Gallan HL, Richards WE, et al. Laparoscopy during pregnancy: a study of laparoendoscopic surgeons. *J. Reprod. Med.* 1997;42:33-8.
[83] Moreno-Sanz C, Pascual-Pedreno A, Picazo-Yeste JS, Seoane-Gonzalez JB. Laparoscopic appendectomy during pregnancy: between personal experiences and scientific evidence. *J. Am. Coll. Surg.* 2007;205:37–42.
[84] Reedy MB, Kallen B, Kuehl TJ. Laparoscopy during pregnancy: a study of five fetal outcome parameters with use of the Swedish Health Registry. *Am. J. Obstet. Gynecol.* 1997;177:673–9.
[85] Lachman E, Schienfeld A, Voss E, et al. Pregnancy and laparoscopic surgery. *J. Am. Assoc. Gynecol. Laparosc.* 1999;6:347–51.
[86] Friedman JD, Ramsey PS, Ramin KD, Berry C. Pneumoamnion and pregnancy loss after second trimester laparoscopic surgery. *Obstet. Gynecol.* 2002;99:512–3.

[87] Affleck DG, Handrahan DL, Egger MJ, Price RR. The laparoscopic management of appendicitis and cholelithiasis during pregnancy. *Am. J. Surg.* 1999;178:523-9.
[88] Shaefer C. Drugs during pregnancy and lactation. 1st ed. The Netherlands: Elsevier; 2001.
[89] Barnes SL, Shane MD, Schoemann MB, Bernard AC, Boulanger BR. Laparoscopic appendectomy after 30 weeks pregnancy: report of two cases and description of technique. *Am. Surg.* 2004;70:733-6.
[90] Levin DL. Morphologic analysis of the pulmonary vascular bed in infants exposed in utero to prostaglandin synthetase inhibitors. *J. Pediatr.* 1978;92:478–83.
[91] Moise KJ, Huhta JC, Sharif DS, et al. Indomethacin in the treatment of premature labor: effects on the fetal ductus arteriosus. *N. Engl. J. Med.* 1988;319:327–31.
[92] Alano MA, Ngougmna E, Ostrea Jr. EM, Konduri GG. Analysis of nonsteroidal antiinflammatory drugs in meconium and its relation to persistent pulmonary hypertension of the newborn. *Pediatrics.* 2001;107:519–23.
[93] Rumack CM, Guggenheim MA, Rumack BH, Peterson RG, Johnson ML, Braithwaite WR. Neonatal intracranial hemorrhage and maternal use of aspirin. *Obstet. Gynecol.* 1981;58(Suppl):52S–6S.
[94] Corby DG. Aspirin in pregnancy: maternal and fetal effects. *Pediatrics.* 1978;62:930–45.
[95] Major CA, Lewis DF, Harding JA, Porto MA, Garite TJ. Tocolysis with indomethacin increases the incidence of necrotizing enterocolitis in the low-birth-weight neonate. *Am. J. Obstet. Gynecol.* 1994;170:102–6.
[96] Walser HC, Margul.is RR, Ladd JE. Meckel's diverticulitis, a complication of pregnancy. *Obstet. Gynecol.* 1962;20:651-654.
[97] Rudloff U, Jobanputra S, Smith-Levitin M, et al. Meckel's diverticulum complicating pregnancy. Case report and review of the literature. *Arch. Gynecol. Obstet.* 2005;271:89-93.
[98] Cullen JJ, Kelly KA, Moir CR, et al. Surgical management of Meckel's diverticulum. An epidemiologic, population-based study. *Ann. Surg.* 1994;220:564-568.
[99] Tamir IL, Bongard FS, Klein SR. Acute appendicitis in the pregnant patient. *Am. J. Surg.* 1990;160:571-576.

[100] Mahmoodian S. Appendicitis complicating pregnancy. *South Med. J.* 1992;85:19–24.
[101] Machado NO, Grant CS. Laparoscopic appendicectomy in all trimesters of pregnancy. *JSLS.* 2009;13:384-90.
[102] Hee P, Viktrup L. The diagnosis of appendicitis during pregnancy and maternal and fetal outcome after appendectomy. *Int. J. Gynecol. Obstet.* 1999;65:129–135.
[103] Thomas SJ, Brisson P. Laparoscopic appendectomy and cholecystectomy during pregnancy: six case reports. *JSLS.* 1998;2:41–46.
[104] McGory ML, Zingmond DS, Tillou A, Hiatt JR, Ko CY, Cryer HM. Negative appendectomy in pregnant women is associated with a substantial risk of fetal loss. *J. Am. Coll. Surg.* 2007;205:534–540.
[105] Walsh CA, Tang T, Walsh SR. Laparoscopic versus open appendectomy in pregnancy: a systematic review. *Int. J. Surg.* 2008;6:339–344.
[106] Stone K. Acute abdominal emergencies associated with pregnancy. Clin *Obstet. Gynecol.* 2002;45:553–61.
[107] Cappell MS, Friedel D. Abdominal pain during pregnancy. *Gastroenterol. Clin. North Am.* 2003;32:1-58.
[108] Squires RA. Surgical considerations in pregnancy. *Audio Dig. Gen. Surg.* 1998;45:6.
[109] Babler EA. Perforative appendicitis complicating pregnancy. *Am J Med.* Assoc 1908;51:1310-1313.
[110] Kammerer W. Nonobstetric surgery during pregnancy. *Med. Clin. North Am.* 1979;63:1157–64.
[111] Mazze RI, Kallen B. Appendectomy during pregnancy: a Swedish registry study of 778 cases. *Obstet. Gynecol.* 1991;77:835–840.
[112] Al-Fozan H, Tulandi T. Safety and risks of laparoscopy in pregnancy. *Curr. Opin. Obstet. Gynecol.* 2002;14:375–9.
[113] Firstenberg MS, Malangoni MA. Gastrointestinal surgery during pregnancy. *Gastroenterol. Clin. North* Am. 1998;27:73–88.
[114] Masters K, Levine BA, Gaskill HV, Sirinek KR. Diagnosing appendicitis during pregnancy. *Am. J. Surg.* 1984;148:768–771.
[115] Hunt MG, Martin JN Jr, Martin RW, et al. Perinatal aspects of abdominal surgery for nonobstetric disease. *Am. J. Perinatol.* 1989;6:412–417.

[116] Kort B, Katz VL, Watson WJ. The effect of nonobstetric operation during pregnancy. *Surg. Gynecol. Obstet.* 1993;177:371-376.
[117] Punnonen R, Aho AJ, Grönroos M, Liukko P. Appendectomy during pregnancy. *Acta Chir. Scand.* 1979; 145:555-558.
[118] Doberneck RC. Appendectomy during pregnancy. *Am. Surg.* 1985;51:265-268.

Index

A

absorption, 21
acidosis, 21
acute infection, 12
adenitis, 9
agonist, 29
algorithm, 16
alkalosis, 19
alternative hypothesis, 32
analgesic, 25
anatomy, 24
anorexia, 5
antibiotic, 23, 28
antipyretic, 25
anuria, 25
appendectomy, 11, 13, 17, 21, 22, 25, 28, 33, 34, 35, 36, 37, 38
appendicitis, vii, 1, 3, 5, 7, 9, 11, 12, 13, 14, 15, 16, 17, 19, 21, 22, 23, 24, 28, 29, 31, 32, 33, 34, 35, 37, 38
aspiration, 20
asymptomatic, 12
authors, 15, 22, 29

B

bacterial infection, vii
barium, 3
barium enema, 3
bias, 21
birth weight, 22
bleeding, 26
blood flow, 21
bowel, 9, 22, 23, 26
bowel obstruction, 9

C

C reactive protein, vii
carbon, 21, 36
carbon dioxide, 21
carbon monoxide, 21, 36
carcinogenesis, 19
carcinoid tumor, 23
carcinoma, 9
cecum, 4
cholecystectomy, 36, 38
cholecystitis, 9
cholelithiasis, 9, 37
clinical diagnosis, vii, 15, 27
closure, 25
CO_2, 20, 23, 36
colic, 17
color, iv
complications, 20, 21, 24, 26, 28, 32, 35
composition, 14
compression, 23

computed tomography, 34
congenital malformations, 22
consensus, 19
consumption, 27
copyright, iv
CRP, 12
CT scan, vii, 13, 15
cyst, 9

D

damages, iv
data analysis, 28
deaths, 22, 28
defects, 11
dehiscence, 22
delayed gastric emptying, 19
diarrhea, 5
dietary intake, 1
dislocation, 3
displacement, 4, 19, 20
diverticulitis, 9, 25, 26, 37
drugs, 24, 37
ductus arteriosus, 37
dysuria, 5

E

ectopic pregnancy, 9
edema, 19
editors, 35
elaboration, 24
electrocautery, 22
encoding, 14
equipment, 23
evacuation, 15
excision, 26
exposure, 11, 13, 14, 15, 21, 22, 32

F

fat, 15
FDA, 13, 14, 24

fetus, 11, 14, 19, 21, 24, 27, 34
fever, 7
fixation, 4
fluid, 13, 15, 20
Foley catheter, 23

G

gangrene, 1
gastroenteritis, 9
gestation, 24, 29
gestational age, vii, 23, 29
granulocytosis, vii, 12
guidelines, vii, 12, 14, 18, 22
gynecologist, 27

H

harmful effects, 14
heart rate, 23
hematoma, 9
hematuria, 12
hemoglobin, 22
hemorrhage, 37
hernia, 9
hospitalization, 21
hygiene, 1
hypotensive, 20

I

ileum, 26
in utero, 37
incidence, 1, 9, 22, 25, 27, 28, 37
infants, 22, 37
inflammation, 17, 24, 28
inflammatory disease, 9
informed consent, 14
intrauterine growth retardation, 22
intravenously, 23
iodinated contrast, vii, 13

Index

L

lactation, 34, 37
laparoscope, 23
laparoscopic cholecystectomy, 36
laparoscopy, vii, 17, 19, 22, 34, 35, 38
laparotomy, 15, 19, 22, 25, 28
leiomyoma, 28
lesions, 35
leukocytosis, 8, 29
ligament, 9
localization, 4
lower esophageal sphincter, 19

M

magnesium, 29
magnetic field, 14
magnetic resonance, 34
magnetic resonance imaging, 34
management, 19, 27, 31, 32, 34, 35, 37
manipulation, 20, 22, 23
meconium, 37
median, 25
mental retardation, 12
migration, 3
miscarriage, 28
MRI, vii, 13, 14, 15, 33
multiple sclerosis, 31

N

nasogastric tube, 23
nausea, 3, 4
nephrolithiasis, 9
Netherlands, 37
neutrophils, 12
New England, 19

O

obesity, 36
obstruction, 1, 15
omentum, 28
organ, 18
oxygen, 19, 22
oxygen consumption, 19

P

pain, vii, 3, 4, 5, 7, 12, 13, 15, 17, 22, 35, 38
palpation, 7
pancreatitis, 9
pathology, 7, 13, 17, 28, 35
patient care, 34
pelvis, 4, 33
perforation, vii, 7, 12, 15, 23, 24, 25, 27, 29
performance, 14
perinatal, 28, 32
peritoneum, 4, 22
peritonitis, 7, 28
permission, iv
physiology, 35
placental abruption, 9
pneumonia, 9, 15
ports, 23
precursor cells, 12
preeclampsia, 9
pregnancy, vii, 1, 3, 4, 7, 11, 12, 14, 15, 18, 19, 20, 21, 23, 24, 25, 28, 31, 32, 33, 34, 35, 36, 37, 38, 39
prematurity, 12
preterm delivery, 24, 29
proliferation, 11
prophylactic, 23
proteinuria, 12
pulmonary embolism, 9
pulmonary hypertension, 25, 37
pus, 12

R

radiation, vii, 11, 13, 14, 15, 32, 33

Radiation, 11, 15, 32
radiologists, 14
rebound tenderness, vii
recommendations, iv, 11, 13, 14, 21
Registry, 22, 36
relapses, 31
relevance, 12
resection, 26
resources, 34
retardation, 12
rights, iv
risk factors, 29, 33

S

salpingitis, 9
second-generation cephalosporin, 24
sensitivity, 11, 13, 15
sex, 26
sickle cell, 9
signs, vii, 3, 7, 15
Singapore, 35
skin, 23, 24
spontaneous abortion, 12
suppression, 1
surgical intervention, 28
Sweden, 22
symptoms, 3, 4, 5, 15, 17, 29
syndrome, 9

T

tachycardia, vii, 7
temperature, 7, 29
therapy, 28
threatened abortion, 9
thrombosis, 22
time periods, 28
tissue, 22, 36
titanium, 14
torsion, 9, 13
transection, 23
transport, 22
trauma, 22, 28
trends, 1
tumor, 35
tumors, 35
tumours, 13

U

ultrasound, vii, 12, 13, 14, 15, 33
urinary tract, 9
urinary tract infection, 9
urine, 12
uterus, 4, 7, 22, 23, 28

V

vapor, 22
variations, 1
varicose veins, 9
ventilation, 19
vision, 23
vomiting, 3, 4, 15

W

white blood cell count, 12

X

xiphoid process, 23